PRAISE FOR THE

MW00830024

"The *EAT HOT...LOOK HOT*™ diet will save A LOT of women from having to undergo liposuction, the most common plastic surgery procedure in the world."

-Michael Saltzhauer, MD, F.A.C.S. (a.k.a., "Dr. Miami")
Bal Harbour Plastic Surgery Associates, Miami, FL

"Superbly researched and presented in a practical, easy-to-implement manner with plenty of bonus materials and guides, *EAT HOT...LOOK HOT*™ has the power to alter the gold-standard for dieting and permanently transform lives, both physically and psychologically."

-Brad K. Cohen, MD, F.A.C.S., F.A.A.O.S., Surgeon,
Aventura Orthopedics and Sports Medicine, PA, Miami, FL

"As an obstetrician-gynecologist, I care a lot about my patient's way of eating. *EAT HOT......LOOK HOT*™ is a well-researched book that provides an easy way for my patients to stay healthy before, during and after pregnancy. Well done."

-Clones Lans, MD, F.A.C.O.G., Surgeon
Board Certified Obstetrics and Gynecology
Fellow of American College of Obstetrics and Gynecology
Assistant Clinical Professor of Obstetrics and Gynecology
Vice-Chair OBGYN Department Jackson North Medical Center,
Miami, FL

"You're lifted up and you feel better. Trust me people, this is it!"

-Mariela Keen, former *CNN-Español* Consultant;
Owner, *The Juicery Bar,* Miami, FL

"My co-workers noticed, my sister noticed when I saw her Saturday, and I was so excited to tell her that I lost five pounds in one week. And my skin is glowing … and I'm so excited to keep doing the diet because imagine in a month…I'll be able to wear a bikini!"

-Karinis V., Miami, Florida

"I have been traveling the world, and spent two months living in Thailand and Bali, eating the local food. I made no effort to restrict when or what to eat, but I still began to shed pounds. After learning about Alessandra Solis' focused dieting strategy, it became clear to me what occurred, and how to take advantage of this amazing effect."

-Josh Z., Barcelona, Spain

"I'm absolutely loving your book; the research you have done is amazing."

-Susan Housley
Book Reviewer, Midwest Book Review

EAT HOT...
LOOK HOT™

Secret Strategies to Lose Weight Quickly

Burn more Fat and Boost
Your Metabolism at any Age!

SNEAK PREVIEW EDITION

By Alessandra Solis
Creator of EAT HOT...LOOK HOT™

Foreword by Brad K. Cohen, MD, F.A.C.S., F.A.O.O.S

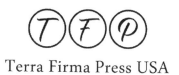

Terra Firma Press USA

Copyright © 2017 by Terra Firma Press USA, Inc.

All rights reserved.

Published in the United States by Terra Firma Press USA, Inc.

12864 Biscayne Boulevard, Suite 119

North Miami, Florida 33181

www.EatHotLookHotDiet.com

Library of Congress Cataloging-in-Publication Data is
Available upon request

ISBN-13:978-0-9991101-9-5

Also available as an eBook

Interior design by Lisa DeSpain
Cover design by C5 Designs
Copyright © Terra Firma Press USA, Inc.
Cover photography by Adobe Stock Premium Collection

10 9 8 7 6 5 4 3 2 1

First Paperback Edition

This book is dedicated to anyone with self-doubt.

It's been said that every journey begins with one step forward. For me, this book that you hold in your hands is the culmination of many of those steps. My advice to you dear readers is to never give up on your hopes and dreams. Forge ahead despite the nagging doubts and naysayers. Believe in yourself and step by step, go confidently in the direction of your dreams.

"One sometimes finds what one is not looking for."
                                    Sir Alexander Fleming,
                                    Discoverer of Penicillin

AUTHOR'S NOTE

Get a Head Start on
Becoming The Sexy New You!

You are about to discover the #1 secret to immediately burn fat, boost your metabolism, literally block further weight gain and upgrade your overall appearance at any age. What's more? There is no exercise component to EAT HOT...LOOK HOT™. It's the star ingredients that trigger quick and dramatic weight loss.

Here is the diet plan in a nutshell, with few caveats:

Eat whatever you typically eat. Just add a little of 'this' and a little of 'that', and voilà, lose weight. It's that simple.

Why? Because this revolutionary weight loss plan, backed by ground-breaking scientific research that I will show you, relies only on 'additions' and not on 'subtractions'.

True or False?
- To lose weight, I need to consume less calories
- To burn off excess fat, I must either eat less or exercise more
- All diets require giving up something
- Long-term weight loss success requires significant change and effort

- Dieting will leave me hungry and deprived, one way or another
- Before I can lose weight, I must first figure out what caused my weight gain to begin with, and address its cause

If you answered 'True' to any of the statements above, prepare to be pleasantly surprised as you discover science's latest strategies for rapid, sustainable weight loss.

In order to get *different* results than you have before, you need a *different* approach. That's why you will never need to count calories, fats, carbs or anything else when you follow the EAT HOT... LOOK HOT way of life that originated in swarthy, sexy Miami. You don't need to limit your favorite foods, question why you have been packing on the pounds lately, or omit any food type. It's time to lay all that to rest.

You will just sprinkle in specific ingredients when you are in the mood. The more you decide to sprinkle it in, the hotter you'll start to look!

EAT HOT...LOOK HOT *Sneak Preview Edition* reveals **which additions and combinations** result in a faster metabolism, convert stubborn white fat to the faster burning brown fat, lead you to feel full faster, plus block further weight gain and hinder additional fat deposits. This scientifically-proven diet approach holds the key to dramatic weight loss and to upgrading your overall appearance. Plus, as a side benefit, expect to feel more energized, vibrant and youthful, owing to enhanced blood flow. Men enjoy even greater benefits!

You are about to discover how to boost your metabolism and burn fat at any age by being introduced to the functional ingredients that are the super-star components of the EAT HOT...LOOK HOT diet plan.

So grab your waistline by the hands and get ready for it to look a whole lot smaller!

In this book, **endorsed[1] by physicians and other health professionals,** you will learn:

- How to achieve rapid weight loss and a blocking effect of further weight gain despite eating a high calorie meal

- How to rev your metabolism for hours to come

- What you can eat as an appetizer in order to feel full by the main course

- What to munch on at bedtime if you want to burn *even more* fat while you sleep

- What *not* to eat together with the fat-busting ingredients that will dilute its weight loss and fat-busting effects.

- How long to keep the star ingredient in your mouth before you swallow it, to get faster, more dramatic results.

- Phase Four secret strategies of the EAT HOT...LOOK HOT diet to help you accelerate your results by pairing certain 'additions' together and at certain temperatures.

That is only part of the secret sauce. Discover the rest in the coming chapters.

---

1   All endorsements are unpaid.

Here is a quick glance at just two of the 61 groundbreaking scientific studies that back up the rapid weight loss strategies you will discover in EAT HOT...LOOK HOT.

"Clinical evidence supports a role of *** as an anti-obesity agent. Both oral and gastrointestinal exposure increase satiety and reduce energy and fat intake... [I]t improves lipolysis, increases energy expenditure through the activation of brown adipose tissue in humans... [and] ingestion is associated with an increase in fat oxidation..."

- Leung FW., *Prog Drug Res.* 2014.

"...Taken together, these functional ingredients have the potential to produce significant effects on metabolic targets such as satiety, thermogenesis and fat oxidation."

- Hursel R[2] et. al. *Int J Obes* (Lond). 2010.

Are you tired of feeling heavy and yearn to look as good as you once did?

If so, this book will give you a head-start, nearly an entire year in advance of the full edition's slated release, which includes tailored EAT HOT...LOOK HOT recipes from some of Miami's top chefs, adapted to Phases One through Four of this diet plan. I will take you step-by-step from where you are now to where you want to be.

EAT HOT...LOOK HOT also reveals numerous other world-class scientific studies that show you the specific bodily mechanisms at play causing you to slim down fast. The best part is that you won't even feel like you are on 'a diet' because apart from the 'additions,' you can continue eating as you wish.

Start becoming the sexy new you today! All you have to do is *Eat Hot*...I'll tell you how.

---

2   Department of Human Biology, Nutrition Faculty of Health, Medicine and Life Sciences, Maastricht University, Maastricht, The Netherlands.

FOREWORD

I was initially skeptical when Alessandra Solis asked me to write a foreword for EAT HOT...LOOK HOT™. Could the addition of certain food and spices into one's diet actually promote weight loss in a meaningful way? However, after investigating the matter for myself, I was quite surprised to find that there is actually a large body of research which indeed supports her premise.

In my many years in private practice, I frequently treat obese and overweight patients who have tried and failed at traditional dieting. Their obesity tends to exacerbate common conditions such as high blood pressure, heart disease, lower back pain and arthritis, to note a few. There is now a body of scientific evidence that the traditional approach to dieting, consisting of caloric restriction and activity modification, is ineffective at best, and may actually be harmful. So called yo-yo dieting can lead to additional health problems, depression, and despair. As a result of the caloric restriction, the basal metabolic rate slows down. Even the patients that successfully lost weight on their respective diet tend to regain their lost weight and may end up heavier than before they started dieting. Even worse, their basal metabolic rate remains low, thus making future attempts at weight loss even more difficult.

As a result of chronic hunger and eating bland diet foods, dieters may develop cravings and may actually binge on junk food, further exacerbating their problem. Promoted by the multi-billion dollar diet food industry, "diet foods" in the supermarket are filled with artificial chemicals and ingredients that may actually work against weight loss. Thus, people who diet may be heavier than people who don't diet. Is it therefore any surprise that obesity rates have risen despite the plethora of diets and diet foods available?

Alessandra Solis has compiled a compelling body of evidence that there may be a better way. The addition of the specific food ingredients called for by EAT HOT...LOOK HOT™ has been shown in human and animal studies to speed metabolism, promote abdominal fat loss and curb appetite. Thus, these key ingredients can reverse the typical dieting dilemma. Instead of fighting hunger and a slowed metabolism, readers of EAT HOT...LOOK HOT™ will find a way to lose weight, boost health and enjoy more flavorful food in the process.

I was also quite surprised to find that contrary to popular belief, eating according to Alessandra Solis' novel plan may actually promote gastrointestinal health. There is a body of scientific evidence that over time, these foods can decrease symptoms from dyspepsia (commonly called "heartburn" and "reflux") and actually promote healing of gastric ulcers.

Finally, as Alessandra Solis further elaborates, there are numerous additional health benefits to eating these specific foods. Studies have shown that people on diets with these ingredients may have a lower incidence of heart attack and stroke, lower blood pressure, lower cholesterol and increased blood flow. These ingredients may even boost production of hormones to reduce depression and stress. Further studies have shown that the spices Alessandra Solis recommends may boost immunity and promote longevity. There is even evidence that it can help fight cancer.

In the EAT HOT...LOOK HOT™, Alessandra Solis has presented a fun, easy-to-read, well-organized guide to implement a simple strategy to promote weight loss and health, while avoiding the pitfalls of standard dieting.

- Brad K. Cohen, MD, F.A.C.S., F.A.A.O.S.
Aventura Orthopaedics & Sports Medicine, PA,
Miami, FL

INTRODUCTION

A Tantalizing Taste of the New, Sexy You

I f you're like many other women (and even men), you've tried diet after diet with few lasting results. *So did I.*

So many diets fail because we are just too hungry on them; so when those hunger pangs set in, only the most resolute, strong-willed people can resist the urge to eat. Or perhaps we couldn't keep the weight off because some elements of past diets became too restrictive after a while. It's hard to live with restrictions long-term. Who can keep that up? I couldn't and it's perfectly normal if you couldn't either.

So, what if you tried something entirely new and different? Something that moves away from the soon-to-be passé approach we have all grown up with, which can be summarized as: "Eat less, Exercise more."

That's the diet plan you have right here, one that I created and aptly named EAT HOT...LOOK HOT™. **This rapid weight loss plan only relies on periodically *adding* certain functional ingredients (food, nothing artificial) readily available at the supermarket, that would speed up your metabolism, burn stubborn belly fat, literally block further weight gain by altering activity in your intestines, and make you feel full faster, so you eat less too.** All 'additions' are incorporated in a gradual manner, making it relatively easy to do. This dramatic metabolism-boosting weight loss plan separates this process into Four Phases.

In fact, if you are already committed to (or even trying out) another diet, *Eating Hot* can also be appended to it and will help you adhere to it far more easily, as you will be less hungry and less tempted to "cheat." However, you may want to give up that weight loss plan entirely in favor of a far better, more sustainable approach that does not rely upon restrictions and omissions of any kind. It's an entirely novel approach to weight loss and accelerating your metabolism at any age. While most other diets result in a decreased metabolism, and raise the odds of re-gaining even more weight following the initial loss, EAT HOT...LOOK HOT is expected to have the opposite effect and avoids this pitfall.

While revolutionary in its approach, EAT HOT...LOOK HOT is supported by an abundance of cutting edge scientific research into obesity, weight management, metabolic function, fat oxidation, blood sugar control, and so forth. The studies were largely conducted at world-class medical centers and some reported in the most prestigious of medical journals and nearly all are searchable on PubMed. The medical literature also supports a wide range of health benefits apart from weight loss (or management) when adding these few key ingredients to your existing drinks, meals and snacks.

> "Understand that embarking on a diet that restricts your calories even surreptitiously is a serious gamble with your metabolism."

Fortunately for all of us, because the addition of certain metabolism-boosting foods that are the cornerstones of EAT HOT...LOOK HOT involves only minor adjustments to our existing eating habits, it's very easy to maintain. That means that weight loss no longer needs to be the struggle it once was.

If you were operating under faulty premises before and restricting your calories even surreptitiously, how could you be expected to attain the long-term weight management results you were striving for? That's why this weight loss plan does not restrict your calories but only adds foods with high thermogenic potential that will rev up your metabolism for hours to come and burn unwanted fat. This is a better and easier approach to achieve your goals without backfire later on. Plus there will be no more battles against your body's natural hunger cues. Eat whenever you are hungry.

Are you Ready for The New, Sexy You?

If so, read on. You'll be amazed at the possibilities.

What if simply adding some functional ingredients—which I will call *Hot Foods*—into your regular meals and snacks was enough to change your weight and your life? Imagine that in one month's time, your confidence would soar as your weight decreased, your belly fat melted away, your energy improved, and your skin glowed? Have you given any thought to what this newfound confidence would bring to your life? How much better would you feel about yourself if you thought you had a perfect figure? How happy would you be to take off all that additional weight you've been carrying around?

Beyond weight management, the key foods and spices that comprise the 'additions' that you will be adding into your existing meals, drinks and snacks also happen to confer a wide range of health benefits according to scientific literature. More on that in a later chapter...

This may sound too easy and too good to be true, but what do you have to lose,[3] especially if other approaches were difficult for

---

3   All puns intended. That being said, here is the answer: a lot of weight and extra fat!

you to maintain or simply didn't work at all? EAT HOT...LOOK HOT worked for me and others who have eaten this way—and it should work for you too. Best of all, it doesn't require much overhaul to what you are doing *right now*. EAT HOT...LOOK HOT mostly just involves adding certain foods containing the key functional ingredients to your existing meals and snacks, and it is no matter if your existing meals consist of pasta or a hamburger and your preferred snack food is a big bag of potato chips.

In fact, if you like potato chips, you will be at a significant advantage as far as this diet goes—especially if you like to eat *a lot* of potato chips. *What?* I can imagine your reaction as you re-read that last sentence. Just read forward now, not backwards; and soon you will understand why.

By now, you probably realize that EAT HOT...LOOK HOT is revolutionary in its approach. It's unlike any other diet plan I have ever heard of because you will not need to deprive yourself of anything that you want to eat or would normally eat—not even cookies. No counting calories, fat, carbs, or anything else, for that matter. This plan does not require you to stop eating for emotional comfort, in times of stress, anxiety or boredom. In fact, that might be a good way to schedule in the *Hot Foods* as a snack.

To lose weight, you simply *add* certain *Hot Foods* that I will gradually introduce you to. Even if you don't "like" spicy food right now, don't worry: in a few weeks' time (especially with my four-phase approach to acclimating your taste buds to these add-ons), you will become so accustomed to it that the heat shouldn't bother you anymore. Plus, you will look so terrific that eating this way will be a miniscule price to pay for all the benefits coming your way. It's worth repeating: even if you don't like spicy foods, can only tolerate a drop of spice, or never ate anything spicier than a graham cracker, you can still dramatically lose weight following this diet plan with small, incremental changes. Besides, if you are not already acclimated to the star ingredients that I introduce and incorporate **gradually** in this diet plan, you will likely have an **even more dramatic response** to a lesser amount of spice when you first start out. (*Author's Note*: People used to *Eating Hot* may have to begin the diet at Phase Three to see dramatic results, or take care **not to simultaneously eat the two main foods that dilute the weight management effects of the star ingredients**, that you will learn about later in the book. Spicy eaters can also pair the different *Hot Foods* to get a synergistic effect, such as adding ginger or green tea to existing spicy meals.)

As you build your tolerance as you move through the Four Phases of EAT HOT...LOOK HOT, you will not think that the earlier tiny amounts of the star ingredients taste like much of anything anymore, and you might even find yourself looking forward to adding more *Hot Foods* because you are no longer used to eating bland. All the while, you will start to look better and better if you are consuming the 'additions' and not diluting their effects by pairing it with the two main foods that I will warn you about later in the book.

If after a month on the diet you decide that you are tired of eating the *Hot Foods*, you can always walk away with your radical weight loss in one month's time (around 18 pounds, if you follow this plan as written)—and still walk away a winner. It's kind of like the game shows where you see someone reach a certain reward level and then, with trepidation, they quit before winning the million dollars because they feel that they've had enough. They still walk away with a prize ... just not the grand prize...

If you are still hesitant to begin, think of it as though you are entering a competition which you can quit at any time or resume at any time, and that you get to keep the prizes you gained during "play time", so it's a winning proposition.

Some people seem afraid of change (but I'm sure you've heard the Chinese joke concerning the definition of "insanity", right? If not, here it is: Doing the same thing but expecting a different result.)

Others with heartburn or ulcers have wondered out loud if *Eating Hot* could have any ill effect (yes, it can, according to reflux expert, Dr. Jonathan Aviv, whom I interviewed for this book, so if you suffer from GERD, this is not the diet for you.) Other people seem to be plagued by emotional road-blocks. If you can relate to these psychological barriers, before you think to yourself, "I can't do this" and sabotage your opportunity here, work on changing your thoughts to a positive mindset and visualize all the benefits of slimming down and proudly showing off your new figure.

You can do it! Before you know it, you may be hitting the "I'm a Success Story" button on the website to be our feature story of the month, and submitting *Before* and *After* photos chronicling your big success! In fact, our monthly winner can look forward to many exciting bonuses and prizes. Winners will be announced at the beginning of each month on the website (and in the newsletter sign-up for the latest happenings) starting February 2018, so stay tuned and inspired...In fact, I want you to take your *Before* photo today, and save it. Mark the date. I want you to take an *After* photo every month thereafter that you are on my EAT HOT... LOOK HOT plan. Document your progress; when it is dramatic and you have the results you want, send it in! I want to hear from you (click the Testimonials tab on the website) and send photos of your dramatic transformation.[4] Or click the big "I'm a Success Story!" button.

---

4   By submitting your results, you grant Terra Firma Press USA, Inc. and this author permission to use your name, photos and testimonials in connection with their publicity efforts on behalf of the EAT HOT...LOOK HOT diet.

You will be astonished at just how easy this weight loss plan is. You control the pace and how spicy or not-so-spicy you make some of your meals and snacks.

I almost forgot to tell you this important part up front: EAT HOT...LOOK HOT does not even have an exercise component! In fact, I didn't even realize that I was on "a diet," or why I was losing weight and looking better all around. This is how it all happened...

CHAPTER ONE

SERENDIPITY LED ME INTO AN EFFORTLESS DIET THAT REALLY WORKS!

L et me tell you how it all happened:

As you may have guessed already, this diet was an accidental discovery.

Like many other great breakthroughs that are discovered seemingly by happenstance, the origin of EAT HOT...LOOK HOT was a total fluke that had the unexpected happy outcome of slimming down in a short period of time in a nearly effortless way. I wasn't trying to lose weight or get in shape, and I certainly wasn't thinking about writing a book on anything; let alone on weight loss. After all, I was a somewhat pudgy mother of two in my early forties planning a 125-person family reunion, all while trying to get rid of a cold. Pretty mundane, right?

In fact, the story I am about to share with you was no less than a godsend. My sole objective was to de-congest and do what I could to counter the frequent colds I was catching so that I could feel well enough to enjoy this important weekend-long affair that I had spent a few months planning and really looking forward to. It was the biggest family event I had planned since my wedding many years prior.

Between my little daughter in kindergarten and my husband's work in an emergency room in Miami during the busy flu season,

I seemed to catch one upper respiratory virus after another, and no amount of Purell seemed to change this. My doctor would joke that whatever germs my kids didn't bring home from school, my husband—who was exposed to all sorts of viruses in the ER, given that Miami is a winter hot spot for tourists—would contribute, just to fill in any gaps.

I was congested and sluggish, and desperately wanted to feel well enough for the weekend affair that was fast approaching, the following month. I knew from past experience that my colds just linger on and on, sometimes leading to a sinus infection, and it seemed that one didn't go away completely before the next one began.

I suddenly eyed my son's bag of Sweet and Spicy Jalapeño Potato Chips in the pantry, recalling one particular day in my early 20s (which was 20 years ago and counting) when my friend, unbeknownst to me, put some chili pepper flakes on my pizza. When I took my first bite ever of spicy food, I was somewhat stunned because not only did my mouth feel the heat, but my eyes and nose started running profusely. I wasn't quite sure what was happening. And then something wonderful followed, all those years ago: my head felt amazingly clear, my sinuses opened, and I felt great, despite the fact that it was hay fever season in New York, which typically left me congested for about six weeks straight.

I had not braved spicy food since then—at least, not intentionally. Once I had a tad of spicy Indian food for a work engagement, which mostly ended up in my napkin. Now fast-forward from my 20s back to my present early 40s, with my stuffed nose and head, eyeing my son's potato chips bag with its big red SPICY warning sign plastered on the packaging. *Maybe I'll give this another try*, I thought to myself. I really needed relief and I was desperate, praying to be well. I had a big guest list, people coming in from out of town, back-to-back events for three days at three different venues with three different caterers, and there was no event planner.

I was running the whole show—all three of them, actually. For all my pain-staking work and all the debt we were incurring to host this weekend-long event, I wanted to fully enjoy it and not feel sick and tired and stuffed up—my usual state of being since my son had entered nursery school ten years before.

Ironically, my son knows me all too well and knows I'll snack on his food while he is at school, so he'd purposely bought spicy chips, thinking that I wouldn't touch them because he knows I don't like spicy food. Well, he was wrong. I really wanted to feel better, so I decided to brave those chips. I started munching on them, and fought the urge to grab a piece of bread to dilute the spice. I wanted my nose to run: the more, the better. I reveled in un-stuffing my nose and head and feeling relief that lasted hours! If I had to eat jalapeño chips for five weeks to feel good during the busy final planning stages for the reunion and to partake in all the festivities, then so be it, even if it wasn't my taste. Feeling better was all that mattered to me. Of course, losing 10 or 15 pounds would have been nice too, but that hadn't been happening, and I took it off my radar. I was resigned to the fact that maintaining an ideal weight after 40 poses a formidable challenge I didn't think I could beat without practically starving myself or doing a lot of exercise. I had no interest in either of those options.

In fact, I had previously been trying to diet for months on and off, and all I had to show for it (with only about a month left to the reunion) was further weight gain! It was rather disheartening.

Once I turned 40, like most people, I started packing on the extra pounds, and I am not really sure why. Of course, I would've liked to lose some of those if possible—but it seemed that my metabolism had slowed and it was getting harder to lose weight and easier to gain it. I was going to turn 43 the day after the last party, and at that point, I was ready to settle for "not looking fat," even if that meant that I didn't look slim, either. As for "looking hot," that I assumed was out of the question. My 20s were long over. Even my 30s were.

So I bought a maxi-cut dress to conceal some midriff fat, and hoped the aqua blue stones positioned not far from my face would draw the eye there and not to the enlarged hips further south.

Then something remarkable and unexpected happened: each week, I started getting slimmer and slimmer without dieting or changing anything else about my life. I was (happily) baffled. I was eating cookies, pizza, pasta, meat and potatoes, and hadn't "dieted" for even a single day, yet I was losing, losing, losing...With a 15-pound weight loss in a month (I lost more like 17 pounds, but I had a little over a month to do so), people were taking notice. *I* was taking notice.

By the time I was ready to get the final tailoring done on my maxi dress—which I didn't even belong in anymore—it was at least one size too big on me. I had slimmed down from 138 lbs. on a good day, to a sexy 121 pounds (I am on the tall side, so that is really thin for me) in just under five weeks! My family and friends couldn't understand how I had gotten so slim.

The truth was, neither did I.

My husband and I went on vacation to New York the following month of January, and there I started pondering how I'd lost the weight that I seemed to be slowly gaining back. I asked myself— *what was I doing then that I'm not doing now?*

That's when it dawned on me: I had stopped trying to fight my colds (in anticipation of the reunion weekend) with those jalapeño potato chips. I then wondered if jalapeño could promote dramatic weight loss. I had never heard of that before. So I turned to *Google's* handy search engine on my iPhone, and lo and behold, the answer was an astonishing *yes*! I suddenly realized that if I wanted to keep *looking* hot, I would have to continue *eating* hot.

It was then and there, on a cold, snowy night in our hotel room in Manhattan's trendy Upper West Side, that the basic premise for EAT HOT...LOOK HOT was born, and this book is aptly named for that premise. It's been almost three years since then an in that time, I have delved into solid scientific literature backing what I had individually experienced. I then presented my diet plan to a couple of physicians who I asked to look into the scientific bases of my revolutionary diet plan. After getting (all unpaid) endorsements and the green light, I focused on devising an incremental diet plan (beyond just eating jalapeño potato chips in a haphazard way) with meal plans and recipes to accompany it, that I could share with the world. I was energized by thinking that if I went ahead with this book, I would be able to help so many other people struggling to keep their weight down.[5] I was amazed just thinking about the vast number of people that could be offered such an easy way to lose weight, and all the great benefits that that bestows. The weight loss process was so easy, in fact, that I hardly even noticed that I was eating much differently. Realizing the benefit I could bring to other people was exhilarating: I felt like I suddenly had a new mission in life.

From Then to Now

I have spent the past three years researching scientific study after study that have elucidated for me how to craft a diet plan from that big clue I got around the time of the reunion. I've taken the diet far beyond jalapeño potato chips. Besides, when it comes to the star ingredient that leads to dramatic effects on your metabolism, not all potato chips are created equal!

---

5   Neither this diet nor any other diet program should be followed without first consulting a healthcare professional. If you have any special conditions, are pregnant, nursing or have any medical condition requiring attention, or if you take medication or supplements, you should consult your healthcare professional regularly regarding initiation and possible modification of the program contained in this book. The author, endorsers and publisher expressly disclaim any responsibility for any adverse effects that may result from use or application of the information contained in this book.

With the added time, experimentation and after pouring over the newest scientific research together with other physicians, I came to understand the various mechanisms at play that result in quick, dramatic weight loss (and a blocking effect of further weight gain,) and discover that two main food types will negate the fat burning and fat deposit-prevention aspects of eating according to the EAT HOT...LOOK HOT plan, and I warn you about that later in the book. For all my dear readers who want that answer right now, just think about what people eat or drink in haste if they ate something too spicy and want to diminish the hot sensation in their mouth. If you can figure that out, you have your answer; if not, I'll reveal that very soon.

Now, this is very important: if you eat those foods within 30 minutes of consuming the star functional ingredients that are the cornerstone of this diet, the diet will not work well and will barely yield results. That's because the functional ingredients are diluted. The flip side is also true in several ways.

First, eat slowly to maximize how much time the *Hot Foods* are actually *in* **your mouth before swallowing**, since there are certain receptors in the mouth that when activated by these *Hot Foods*, lead you down the road to rapid weight loss. (You can read about it in one of the studies I cite in the *Full Edition*.)

These receptors are activated when a key chemical substance contained in certain foods that are part of EAT HOT...LOOK HOT are actually present in your mouth, activating these receptors. As such, try *not* to eat quickly, but wait until the hot feeling in your mouth subsides before taking the next bite. A quick rule of thumb: Let your nose start to run before you take the next bite. **This will maximize your weight loss and will speed up your metabolism even further.** The diet still works whether you eat at a regular pace or not; this is just a method to get even more dramatic results and to minimize how much *Hot Foods* you need to eat, in the event that it is not yet your taste.

If you combine different super-star ingredients featured in EAT HOT...LOOK HOT, you amplify the weight loss effects. Even eating the *Hot Foods* together with warm or hot tea, hot (or warm) soup or anything else heated up will amplify the effects of the key functional ingredients that you will be consuming on this plan. If you can add some black pepper or ginger to your warm soup, you can absolutely call it a Phase Four Meal!

More on this when we get to Phase Four of the diet plan.

EAT HOT...LOOK HOT IS *NOT* A LOW-CALORIE DIET IN DISGUISE

Now, this is *not* a low calorie diet in disguise. Most other diets are just that. Experts agree that in time, a low calorie diet will SLOW your metabolism after the initial weight loss period despite following the diet to a T. Most people relate that, at best, they plateau but cannot return to their pre-diet caloric intake without getting even fatter than they originally were, and hence are stuck forevermore eating less, being hungry and deprived or accepting a heavier version of their pre-dieting selves. Not great no matter how you slice it! When looked at through this prism, understand that embarking on a diet that restricts your calories even surreptitiously is a serious gamble with your metabolism. So we are definitely not falling for that trap and you will never, ever count or limit your calories or fat on this diet.

That's another reason EAT HOT...LOOK HOT sets itself apart from all of the other diets lining the shelves of bookstores. You will actually end up eating more calories on most days, yet you will rev your metabolism up very naturally to burn off even more than you take in—by a long shot. I also have a method for burning extra fat even while you sleep. While most people's metabolism are slower in the evenings, if you do one simple thing, like snack on a handful of special potato chips at bedtime, you should weigh in even thinner come morning. It's not just any potato chip; most will result in weight gain. I'll tell you in a later chapter which ones work best, if at all.

That is what this diet is all about. It gives readers an effortless way to reach and maintain an ideal weight without feeling hungry and deprived. The approach of EAT HOT...LOOK HOT is revolutionary in that you will mainly be adding certain foods and spices to your meals and snacks instead of subtracting certain categories of food (depending on what diet you would otherwise be trying) out of your diet.

> **Enjoy life, just make it a little spicier.**
>
> *That's your new motto; repeat it to yourself 5 times a day for added success. Don't forget to implement it too whenever you feel like it, preferably 5 times a day. If that means you eat 3 hearty fattening meals a day, that's okay, as long as you snack on one of the foods I highlight in this book about 5 times a day, when the mood strikes.*

Since, as I mentioned in the Introduction, EAT HOT...LOOK HOT does not have an exercise component, you can sleep in and still burn off your excess fat. Especially if you eat certain thermogenic (metabolism boosting) food right before bed... Word of caution: Don't eat potato chips at bedtime or during the day until you understand which work and why. Otherwise, you'll gain rather than lose!

Remember, this diet plan is all about additions, never subtractions. It's a fat-busting, metabolism-speeding diet with many health benefits, but common sense dictates that some of those added health benefits might be mitigated if your net diet is unhealthy. Bear in mind though, this is not primarily a book on how to attain a balanced, healthy diet; this is a weight loss book to get you looking and feeling *Hot*.

It's up to you what else you eat in addition to the metabolism-boosting, fat-burning foods that are the bedrock of EAT HOT... LOOK HOT.

EAT HOT...LOOK HOT Can Be Appended to Almost Any Other Diet You Are Already Committed To

There is no diet plan I have ever heard of which is this simple and flexible, yet offers quick and effective results that will last as long as you continue incorporating specific foods into your diet. One of the many benefits of this diet plan in terms of its flexibility is that it can be applied to and appended to many other diets. If you are already on or committed to a certain diet plan, such as a gluten-free diet, vegan, vegetarian, kosher, or even the Paleo Diet, just to name a few, you would simply apply the principles of EAT HOT...LOOK HOT to your existing way of eating in order to lose weight, burn fat, feel full faster, and block further weight gain.

Stop and Start Again Anytime You Want

There is not even an issue if you stop the diet altogether, if you want a break (although don't expect to lose weight during those times, obviously.) You might gradually gain back some of the weight if you are consuming more calories than you are burning, but you can periodically do "tune ups"—say, after gaining back a few pounds—and quickly lose weight again. That's what I do, and it works great for me. This way, I can eat any of the creamy dishes at my favorite Italian restaurants without guilt, even on days when I am not following this diet plan at all. Now, even when I splurge during holiday season and gain a few pounds, it is *no big deal* anymore (like it used to be) and the weight gain is no longer emotionally distressing for me because I know it is not permanent weight gain that will be hard to address down the road.

It's the opposite, now. It's so easy to take off the extra pounds that it is *no big deal* if I gain a few pounds temporarily if I feel like abandoning the EAT HOT...LOOK HOT eating plan for whatever reason. When I am ready to lose weight, I just eat those jalapeño potato chips or other spicy fare throughout the day for the next week and a half and voilá, I am back to my slim self all over again.

Before you think to yourself *Got it*, and put this book down, I must tell you that not all jalapeño potato chips are created equal. Some are quite spicy and really rev things up and some aren't. Also, they cannot be eaten with milk (except non-fat milk) or bread or you risk diluting the active functional ingredient, capsaicin. Milk fats and dairy products that are not fat-free contain casein, a compound that binds with capsaicin oil and then washes it away. It's not that you need to give up dairy on this diet; you can eat or drink it at any time other than right before or after you consume something with capsaicin, in order to get the full metabolism boosting effect. I think 30 minutes before and after is a safe bet.

Run a personalized experiment at home:

Eat something spicy and let it stay in your mouth until it feels hot, for about 30 seconds. In the first of these personalized experiments, eat a piece of bread after the 30 seconds lapse and see if that dilutes the burning sensation. Now do the opposite. Repeat, keep the spicy bite in your mouth for 30 seconds and then drink a warm glass of tea. It should feel even spicier once you add the tea. Now repeat, eating the spicy bite of food and keeping it in your mouth for 30 seconds. Then swallow it but rush to drink some cold milk. The heat is diminishing, right? That's because the capsaicin load is being whisked away.

I include tables later on in the book to help guide you, and I'll also disclose **which** potato chips I eat to shed the unwanted pounds. As for the all of the other brands: some are even too hot for me and some are too mild to do much. However, you can think of the not-so-spicy jalapeño chips as warming your palate up to prepare you for the hot stuff—perhaps as an early Phase One approach to adapting to the diet and de-sensitizing your taste buds to these new flavors and hot sensations. However, don't expect much weight change if your food doesn't have enough of the key chemical components inherent in these spices and hot peppers. Additionally, you need to keep in mind that certain foods negate the weight loss effects of the spices while others enhance it, which I will explain in more detail later on. For now, just do not eat milk (or cheese) or bread with the star ingredients, and that is enough to get you started without sabotage.

Men Get Hotter Too!

Hello to all the men out there!! I have some welcome news especially for you: as a side benefit to this diet plan, expect to get hotter in the bedroom too because a star ingredient of **EAT HOT...LOOK HOT gets your blood flowing much better.** (That's why your face gets red with a spicy meal.) Now enjoy the added blood flow in the bedroom as you trim down and get your youthful stamina back up. I have an entire chapter in the upcoming *Full Edition* dedicated just to that.

What's Ahead?

In this book, I'll show you how and why the EAT HOT...LOOK HOT diet plan works, and in the *Full Edition*, I'll take you through four phases of incorporating capsaicin-loaded foods (and not just potato chips) into your meals and snacks. As a bonus, I am including recipes from some of Miami's top chefs for all four phases of the diet in the *Full Edition* due out next year, plus more bonus recipes at the end of the book that can be adapted to any phase of the diet. Some are simple and easy, for those of you who don't want to be bothered much in the kitchen. Other recipes are more complex, created from some of the top chefs in Miami, who were eager to contribute to this book and be part of the EAT HOT...LOOK HOT culture, the greatest diet sensation ever discovered for sustainable rapid weight loss and easy maintenance. The EAT HOT...LOOK HOT diet plan will also leave your skin aglow, owing to the enhanced blood flow triggered by capsaicin-loaded foods.

My hope is that this diet plan will be the answer to your prayers: that it will be *The Diet* to end all diets, offering you the freedom to continue eating everything you enjoy and crave while simultaneously losing all the excess weight and fat that you desire, to help you feel and look your best.

EAT HOT...LOOK HOT has been turning into a *Hot Sensation* in recent months, leading to my decision to release a *Sneak Preview Edition* at a fraction of the full price to give you advanced access to these secret strategies. I would love to hear your feedback, and you can contact me through the website, www.EatHotLookHotDiet.com by clicking on *Submit Feedback* on the drop-down bar.

I am happy to tell you that this program has been endorsed[6] by physicians, a sports medicine expert, and even a famous plastic surgeon who is possibly the most sought-out plastic surgeon in the United States, with a waitlist of nearly two years just to get in the door for the initial consultation. After reviewing this unique diet plan, he said (which would run contrary to his pecuniary interests) that this diet will save A LOT of women from needing liposuction. On top of that and receiving heaps of advance praise from other doctors, book reviewers and foodies, many leading restaurant and hotel chefs have committed to crafting recipes for this EAT HOT...LOOK HOT series, tailored to the Four Phases of this diet plan.

---

6   All physician endorsements are unpaid.

We have lots of fun in store for you too and being that video is so popular these days, the chefs and I will be presenting some of the most sumptuous and fat-busting *hot* recipes and tips on video for your education and entertainment. I plan to insert QR Codes linking to the video in the *Full Edition*, which I am still working on, and in the meantime, I will also be setting up and posting to my own YouTube channel, which you can search for to see what's cooking…and learn from some of the best chefs how to craft made-for-you *Look Hot* recipes.

You are also about to start your own exciting journey, and I assure you, it's not arduous. You just have to get used to eating spicier food and some peppers that I'll discuss throughout the book. I will lead you every step of the way, including how to slowly and incrementally adjust your taste buds. Don't worry if you have never eaten spicy food before or if you don't like it. You only need to eat a little, you'll get used to it and other food will start to taste bland. Plus: it's a small price to pay for how hot, slimmed down and sexy you will look. Especially if in one month, you have become so accustomed to eating this way that some heat in food no longer bothers you, yet you keep looking better, better and even better. Aim to make gradual change in the first weeks and the rest comes easy and is worth it many times over! I speak from personal experience.

Expect to look and feel your hottest all around.

Let's get started…

CHAPTER TWO

THE ESSENCE OF EAT HOT...LOOK HOT, A DIET PLAN EASY TO STICK TO

In the introductory and first chapters, I introduced you to a remarkable way to speed up your metabolism, burn fat and shed unwanted pounds in a very easy and flexible way, but I held back and did not fully reveal the exact secret strategies to lose weight quickly and burn off your unwanted fat. I also alluded to many other side benefits of trying out EAT HOT...LOOK HOT concerning improving your overall health, stamina and appearance, which are all backed by new scientific research. (Longevity can even be added into the better overall health factor!) Now that you can visualize the wide-ranging potentials of this diet plan, you are probably wondering if this is actually attainable and what could be the star ingredient that I keep referring to. It is capsaicin, the active ingredient in chili, salsa, jalapeño, cayenne pepper, and other related peppers. I even found a study that showed weight loss with a non-spicy sweet red pepper that has a similar compound to capsaicin called capsiate, only without the heat. I would reserve that route for someone who just cannot bring themselves to eat spicy fare. I only found one study for the non-spicy red bell pepper, whereas I found study after study for the spicy varieties. In the *Full Edition*, I list many different peppers and their respective heat index.

Building up heat tolerance is a key component of this diet and that is why EAT HOT...LOOK HOT is divided into four phases, gradually becoming hotter and hotter (and so should you!) There is a twist when you get to Phase Four.

Capsaicin, while the star component of EAT HOT...LOOK HOT's phases One through Three, is not the only key weight loss component of this diet, although a very important one. In Phase Four, we will be aiming for a synergistic effect whereby $1 + 1 =$ More than 2. For that, I introduce other functional ingredients such as mustard, tea (especially green tea,) black pepper, ginger, coffee, dairy-free curry mixes and more. Additionally, I pair foods with warm or hot drinks, brews and soups to amplify the spicy fat-busting, metabolism-speeding effects that are the bedrock of this diet.

But first, before you wonder too much about what awaits you when you get to Phase Four of EAT HOT...LOOK HOT, and now that you have an overview of what this diet entails, I would like to expound on just how easy and flexible this diet plan is. Remember: I didn't even realize that I was on "a diet." You may not, either.

EAT HOT...LOOK HOT is a long-term eating plan for weight loss, followed by an easy program to maintain your ideal weight for a lifetime. Why is it so easy? Well, for starters, you won't feel hungry on this diet. Nor will it involve giving up your favorite foods or reducing your portion sizes or calories. Eat whatever you normally eat, do the same activities you normally partake of, and be yourself. There is just one adjustment you will be making: save some appetite for spicy food (in particular, the jalapeños) called for by the EAT HOT...LOOK HOT plan. For those of you who, like I was, are not used to eating spicy fare, the heat does take a month or two to get used to. But as the pounds effortlessly melt away to reveal a sexier, slimmer version of you, you will be glad you added the peppers. The Latinos don't call sexy ladies *"Hot Tamales"* for nothing!

Skip trying to find what's to blame for those extra pounds: toxins, hormones, menopause, lack of exercise, allergies, eating wrong for your blood type or eating too many carbs or too much fat or eating the wrong carbs or the wrong fats. The modern-day list of culprits goes on and on. Just look in any bookstore's diet section and you will see them all.

The EAT HOT...LOOK HOT plan is completely different. You can keep doing everything you're doing, even if it's "all wrong", and still lose weight! Just add some ground cayenne pepper, tabasco sauce, jalapeños and other capsaicin-loaded foods and call it a success!

To the seasoned dieter, this might sound too good to be true; or like some kind of gimmick. To understand the science behind this diet and why it works, I have dedicated several scientific chapters (along with references) to explain how eating certain foods that contain capsaicin, the active ingredient of chili peppers, causes weight loss/weight management through several distinct mechanisms. As an added benefit for those concerned with excess belly fat, one of those mechanisms burns belly fat which, in and of itself confers a wide range of health benefits, according to the latest research studies. Another study (which you will read about in the following chapter) showed that white belly fat (which, the study authors explain, is much harder to burn) was transformed into brown belly fat (the kind that is easier to burn and get rid of) after the consumption of capsaicin-loaded food.

So many diets fail because we are just too hungry on them; so when those hunger pangs set in, only the most resolute, strong-willed people can resist the urge to eat. With the EAT HOT... LOOK HOT diet plan, since you can eat whenever you want in amounts that satiate you and can enjoy all the comfort foods that taste and feel so good, you don't feel deprived. There is no need to give up your favorite foods in order to lose weight. Just by adding chili peppers, you are revving up your metabolism to burn off extra calories for hours to come, diminishing your appetite for hours going forward and accelerating the metabolism of lipids (fats.)

Here is your typical dieting scenario: Amy, a five-foot-two inch woman, wants to lose weight and goes on a diet, restricting her calories to 1100 per day. She is very hungry, but manages to keep it up for two and a half weeks, and loses a few pounds. Then Amy's willpower dissipates and she returns to her usual 2,000-calorie-a-day diet. What happened to her metabolism during those two and a half weeks of calorie restriction? According to the editors of *Prevention*[7], her metabolism slowed in response to the body's innate protection from starvation. She was still burning enough calories to lose weight while eating 1100 calories a day, perhaps, but now her daily caloric allowance likely went from 1800 calories a day to less than that. When she resumes eating the way she did in the past, regretfully, she gains back even more weight due to her newly-slowed metabolism.

Amy was in a "Catch 22" situation.

What is unique about EAT HOT...LOOK HOT is that you avoid Amy's predicament and accelerate your metabolism while losing weight, instead doing the opposite!

It is especially helpful to eat foods containing jalapeño in its spice form when snacking (and especially, adding a bedtime snack of spicy potato chips), as this will keep up your metabolism rate while you are asleep. Normally the metabolism slows during sleep, but when you eat foods at bedtime containing jalapeño or their related peppers, you can look forward to a flatter stomach when you wake up in the morning.

---

7   Based on "Metabolism-Boosting Food Rules," by Dan Benardot, PhD, RD, and Associate Professor of Nutrition and Kinesiology at Georgia State University, and Tammy Lakatos, RD.

And now for the Big Reveal:

Which spicy potato chip was behind my initial dramatic weight loss that I told you about in Chapter One?

The Answer: Cape Cod's *Sweet and Spicy Jalapeño Potato Chips*[8]

Since then, though, I must say that I also use other brands as this one is not always in-stock or available where I shop. Some seem better than others for weight loss. I will include a table in the *Full Edition* to guide you phase-by-phase.

Remember: this diet is only about 'additions.' It's worth repeating, since it's not what you would expect to hear from your typical weight-loss diet plan: *There is no need to subtract anything that you want to eat or would normally eat.* To lose weight, you must *only* add hot foods. It is truly revolutionary in its approach, unlike any other diet plan ever created.

EAT HOT...LOOK HOT separates this process into four distinct phases designed to help you integrate these types of foods slowly into your diet as you adjust to the spicy hot flavor (which is somewhat uncomfortable at first for people who are not used to eating hot food). The recipes in the *Full Edition* that accompany each of the four phases of EAT HOT...LOOK HOT will gradually ease you into this eating plan, presenting a wide range of dishes that are easy to prepare. They hold illustrations of simple ways to incorporate jalapeños and other capsaicin-loaded foods into the dishes that you normally prepare, sending you on a culinary tour of some of the best dishes offered by top Miami chefs, who contributed to the recipe section of this book.

The quick and dramatic results of this diet will give you a sense of encouragement—even if spicy foods are not exactly what your taste buds prefer—when you hear so many people complementing

---

8 My favorite brand, and the one I snacked on before the reunion that caused my dramatic weight loss. It's pretty spicy!

you on how slim you look, how great you look, or how much younger you look. When you can wear lingerie and not feel self-conscious about sporting extra pounds, you will sense that your significant other is literally hot to trot!

The results of the EAT HOT...LOOK HOT program are quick and dramatic because the core mechanisms of weight loss work in an additive fashion. Several of the chapters that follow delve into the scientific mechanisms at work, for those who want to learn more. However, the important point here is that, when following this plan daily, peppering your meals (or at least some snacks throughout the day) with jalapeño, cayenne or any of the related spicy peppers (the operative word here is *throughout*. You want to keep your metabolism running high throughout the day and into the night), you can expect to lose upwards of half a pound a day. That's about what I lost. Before discovering this phenomenon, I had felt a dip in my metabolism resulting in a dreaded slow and steady weight gain, beginning when I turned 40. Losing a half a pound a day is 15 pounds in a 30-day month. It was incredible; and best of all, it was effortless! I couldn't believe my good fortune in stumbling upon this like I did. It is truly my pleasure to now spread that good fortune and share these strategies with you.

When I first thought about sharing this wonderful diet plan with others in the months following my dramatic weight loss, I kept thinking it could be the answer to so many people's yearnings to lose weight. Americans are known, as a society, to struggle with weight issues and obesity. People desperately want to lose weight and look great again. EAT HOT...LOOK HOT just seemed to be the perfect diet even for those people who'd failed at other diets. That is because you can still eat and drink the food that you have been eating and drinking all along, even when you would typically gain weight. There is no need to say *goodbye* to your favorite cookie. That is true beauty of EAT HOT...LOOK HOT.

You will never *feel* deprived because you won't *be* deprived of any food or drink that you want. That's what makes this diet plan easy to stick with. As long as you consistently add a few bites here and there of spicy, capsaicin-loaded food (a detailed plan for a slow, systematic introduction is included in the *Full Edition*, along with tasty recipes that you can easily throw together), you *will* lose weight. This plan also differs from other popular diet plans in that you do not have to eat certain foods on certain days or think about the ratios of carbs, proteins or fats; nor do you need to exclude a certain food group, like carbohydrates. Best of all, there is no counting calories (or anything else) on this diet. There are no 5:30 AM alarm bells ringing to goad you to the gym.

Your mind can relax.

What is also so spectacular is that if you don't like to cook, you can skip most of the recipes. Just add hot sauce to your dishes, have salsa with your corn chips, and buy jalapeño-spiced potato chips at the supermarket, and you will lose the weight just the same. It happened to me and will most likely happen to you if you give EAT HOT...LOOK HOT a try for one month. In all practicality, you will see a difference in two weeks; but I say "a month" because it is such a happy feeling to go down at least a whole dress size (which usually correlates to 12 pounds). This will take about three and a half weeks if you follow the plan outlined in this book.

While exercising is a worthwhile daily activity and confers a wide range of health benefits completely separate from losing or maintaining weight, it is not a necessary component of this plan, as far as weight loss or maintenance is concerned. The focus of this book is not about obtaining optimal health—although adding these functional ingredients have been tagged in numerous scientific articles and studies as being particularly healthy to consume.

This is primarily a book for people who want to lose weight, look more radiant, and start to drop jaws (or, at least, look more sleek and slimmed down.) This book is also geared for individuals who want to avoid the dreaded weight gain to begin with. It is way of eating for people who want to *Look Hot*.

On that *hotness* note, that's the way of life here in Miami. This city is heavily populated and influenced by Latin and South American culture; one that values looking sexy, youthful, and sleek for as long as possible, even into the later decades of life. When you live in a city that calls for wearing a bikini year-round, no one here can afford to wait a few months for noticeable weight loss to occur.

If EAT HOT...LOOK HOT is followed properly and consistently, you can expect to drop down about one dress size per month without adding an exercise component. It's no wonder EAT HOT...LOOK HOT has become a *Hot Sensation* (all puns intended). Eat what you want, when you want—just add a few bites, every few hours, of food containing one of the featured chili peppers or its powder, and call it a "weight-loss day." Simple, yes; but true? Absolutely!

Just think of Latinas: they tend to eat spicy foods quite a bit. Look how good American actress and businesswoman Eva Longoria looks, for example. She told *Health*: "My most requested thing to cook for friends is Mexican tortilla soup, guacamole and chili-rubbed skirt steak." Eva is not participating in or endorsing the EAT HOT...LOOK HOT diet; but given the types of spicy foods she loves to make, she's reaping the benefit of a taste for her Mexican-American heritage's peppery dishes and their healthy impact. Selena Gomez's once revealed that her favorite snack included *Hot Cheetos*, for another example.

Some say variety is the spice of life. Since you will be adding quite a bit of spice, let's aim for some variety. It's not necessary, but this will keep things interesting, and you will be more likely to stick with the plan. That's why I include plenty of recipe suggestions in the *Full Edition*.

As I wrote in the introductory remarks, I stumbled upon this realization by accident, when I was desperate to fight the constant colds I was catching during the winter season. As the weeks and then days neared to the big weekend-long event, I made sure to eat those jalapeño-spiced potato chips not only throughout the day, but especially before bedtime. I diligently ate a handful before bed because I knew that when the body sleeps, it repairs itself and fends off viruses and infections.

Later on, when I started to research the magic behind the jalapeño and related foods, I found research studies suggesting that these spicy peppers do fight colds and flus. I wasn't sure if it just was acting like a decongestant or if it actually went after the cold virus, but my research since then strongly implies that the active ingredient in chili peppers does in fact fight viruses and infections, as an added benefit to weight management—a fact which was discussed in detail in those medical journals. I also noticed research that shows that jalapeños and habaneros (another hot pepper) have a slew of other health benefits, which I expound upon in an upcoming chapter. To make a long story short: not only will you keep your weight down, but you will probably also feel better and have increased energy. Who doesn't feel better without a brewing cold?

Not to mention the biggie here: how nice will it be to finally be able to say goodbye to the era of fad diets in your life and exchange them for a lifelong eating plan that is tailor-made for you and by you, as you experiment with which spicy foods to add to your typical diet. I personally can't stand structured eating plans, like that Grapefruit Diet I used to do in high school where I had to eat beets in the afternoon. Do you remember that one? To this day, I gag at the sight of beets.

In contrast, on the EAT HOT...LOOK HOT plan, if you enjoy eating chocolate chip cookies with your lunch, it's no problem. Pizza? Fine. If you can toss some spicy pepper flakes on top of your pizza, even better, especially during the Phase One acclimation stage where you can still eat cheese with the capsaicin-containing foods.

If that doesn't suit your taste buds, no problem; eat the pizza plain or with whatever toppings you like. All you need to do on the EAT HOT...LOOK HOT plan is to scatter small amounts of spicy food into your meals or snacks whenever and however you want, a few times a day and especially at bedtime. You select which food or beverage gets the spice. The more you do, and the spicier and hotter you can tolerate, the faster you will lose weight. That is why this book is divided into The Four Phases. However, if you are not in a rush and do not have a special occasion you are trying to lose weight for, you can take this eating plan as slow and gradual as you wish and spread it out over a longer period of time.

Some people spend a week on Phase One; especially if they are already used to eating some capsaicin-based food, while others take it more slowly. I would say to give it a month if you are new to *Hot Foods*. However, it's entirely up to you and your comfort zone, keeping your weight loss or maintenance goals in mind coupled with your healthcare provider's recommendations (which are always appropriate to get before starting any new diet.)

By the time you reach Phase Four, you should be ready to intensify the heat sensation and thermogenic action of the diet by consuming the spices and peppers eaten in Phases One through Phase Three together with black pepper, ginger tea, hot green, black or white teas and coffee to amplify the weight loss effects. In addition, you will be spicing up your food to a more intense level after having increased your tolerance for spice.

What I love about this eating plan is that even though I have a knack for cooking (that seems to be a trait I picked up from growing up in a family of gourmet cooks), it is not necessary to cook anything on this plan. I often feel too busy to spend much (or any) time preparing meals that take more than 10 or 15 minutes total from kitchen to table. I noticed, while shopping at *Whole Foods Market* the other day, that there are packaged Indian curries that require only two to five minutes of warming time in a pan (or 90 seconds in a microwave) that are loaded with capsicum, a related compound, along with ginger and other spices. I bought one (and then another, and another...) to try it out, and it was spicy to the tune of my *Phase One* (possibly *Phase Two*) plan. I simply prepared some rice with turmeric, olive oil, salt and pepper for taste, and then heated up the capsaicin-loaded pre-made curry packed in a pouch, combined the two, and voilá: my spicy, fat-busting dinner for the family was complete.

I want to point out at the outset that you should be losing weight and burning fat during Phase One. I lost all my excess weight very quickly and in retrospect, I don't think I ever got past what I have now delineated as Phase One, possibly Phase Two, of my since-created EAT HOT...LOOK HOT diet plan.

Last, but not least, you will see for yourself in the forthcoming chapters that EAT HOT...LOOK HOT is backed by the latest food science research. In fact, as one Board-Certified physician put it after reviewing 61 groundbreaking studies that I presented him with, EAT HOT...LOOK HOT is poised to become the new gold-standard for dieting and weight loss.

All of my weight loss strategies are backed by these revolutionary studies conducted by universities and medical centers around the world and I provide all the citations and what I gleaned from each study I cite in terms of weight management strategies. Researchers have repeatedly flagged capsaicin as an anti-obesity agent.

The *Full Edition*—when it comes out—will give you all the tools you need so that you can start and stop at any time. Taking a break from *Eating Hot* is not a problem on this unique plan. You can always resume the EAT HOT...LOOK HOT plan at a later date and have everything you need to resume losing weight once again. This *Sneak Preview Edition* will give you many important tools to get you started to quick and easy weight loss, and as soon as it's ready, in the EAT HOT...LOOK HOT *Full Edition*, I will give you all the rest: from the scientific studies, the gradual acclimation schedule of the Four Phases, all of the meal suggestions and specific meal plans, and the "Table of Commercially-Packaged Foods" that are suitable *Hot Foods* for each phase of the diet (in case you don't want to cook.) I will also provide you with the "Short-Cut to Weight Loss: Spicy Potato Chips Table" in the *Full Edition* so you can have a better sense of which chips work best for weight loss and is suitable to each phase of this diet plan. Additionally, I am eager to provide you with my specially-tailored recipes for this diet and all of the acclaimed chefs' specially recipes, all of which were carefully adjusted to the Four Phases of EAT HOT...LOOK HOT, and many more resources which will always be at your fingertips. There will be plenty of video and free supplemental material to keep the diet fresh, interesting and a pleasure to be a part of what I believe will be the greatest diet sensation to ever gain traction and keep moving from there.

Most of this material is too intricate for the *Sneak Preview Edition*, but you can read all about it when the *Full Edition* is released next year. Since this is relatively early in my journey as an author and the creator of this fabulous diet plan, I would be thrilled

Bonus Tip:

Introduce capsaicin-containing food early in the meal, even as an appetizer. Since it curbs the appetite once consumed, it should result in less calorie consumption at mealtime.

if any readers would like to become Ambassadors of EAT HOT... LOOK HOT after trying the diet. If so, please contact me through the website, www.EatHotLookHotDiet.com.

Well, I hope you are excited! Remember that this abbreviated edition is just enough to get you started on the journey to becoming the slimmed down, sexy, new you. That being said, I will do my best to include here as many additional tips for weight loss that I can include without sacrificing organization.

So, enough said. Let's get started on the journey to eating hot and looking hotter!

CHAPTER THREE

A BRIEF SCIENTIFIC OVERVIEW

In the Introduction and in Chapters One and Two, you learned about the EAT HOT...LOOK HOT diet plan's weight management potential and the different phases of the diet.

But by now, you are probably wondering exactly how this eating plan results in rapid, sustainable weight loss.

I'll give you the quick answer first, before delving into greater explanations (briefly, in this chapter, and in further detail in the next chapter, where I also cite specific scientific studies demonstrating these mechanisms at play).

Here are the core mechanisms through which capsaicin-loaded foods and spices contribute to weight management:

- Shrinks fat tissues
- Lowers blood fat levels
- Converts white fat to brown fat, which is able to be burned off easier
- Stimulates thermogenesis
- Raises metabolism, including resting metabolism/raises energy expenditure
- Increases fat oxidation

- Reduces appetite. Induces feeling of satiety, so eating less comes naturally.

- Blocks weight gain in mice, even when on a high-fat diet. Prevents weight gain and fat deposits and leads to weight loss.

- Another study in mice supports the contention that dietary capsaicin reduces metabolic dysregulation in obese and diabetic subjects.

Why is it important to learn how to implement EAT HOT...LOOK HOT?

Most Americans are not strangers to the obesity problem that plagues one-third of our population (or even the issue of being "overweight" but not technically "obese," which plagues another third of the population, leaving only one-third of the total population in a healthy weight range.) Yet, with these rates on the rise, most people clearly find this problem a difficult one to solve; if not outright insurmountable. Like the old adage goes: It's so easy to gain, and so hard to lose.

It's not that overweight and even obese individuals don't realize the negative health effects of being overweight. Overweight individuals are just as intelligent as the next person. It's not that they are purposely defying their physician's orders. And it is certainly not the case (as they have been known to be discriminated against) that they have no self-respect and just don't care about their health, appearance, or longevity. Overweight and obese individuals I have spoken with would love a solution to follow that is workable, as opposed to the modern selections: namely, those that will become a battle of willpower versus hunger pangs. People also tend to resist anything overly stringent or complex.

Despite the vast amount of diet books on the shelves, few, if any, provide an easy weight loss plan. In fact, most (if not all) will be radically depriving you of something. What's needed is a new approach—that's where EAT HOT...LOOK HOT differs from any diet you have ever encountered, and that's what you will be learning about throughout the book and beyond. Here, you only add certain foods and spices. And in doing so, see the results for yourself as you effortlessly, and finally, shed those unwanted pounds and transform your appearance.

What about All of the Other Diet Programs to Choose From?

If this problem could be solved by the current diet books lining the shelves of the bookstore or the virtual shelves of Amazon.com, I doubt we would continue to see the rising obesity levels that we see today in America. It's not as if consumers aren't running out to buy them—those aisles are the busy ones!

Nevertheless, recent figures from the Center of Disease Control, citing an abstract from the *Journal of American Medicine*, place the obesity problem among adults in the United States at more than one-third of the adult population.[9] Others estimate the problem to be even more widespread.[10]

Famed physician Dr. Andrew Weil, the Harvard-trained physician who is the founder of the Arizona Center for Integrative Medicine, writes in his *Dr. Andrew Weil's Self-Healing's* Annual Edition that the actual number of obese adults in the U.S. is a whopping 62%.[11] A recent article in *Time Magazine*[12] that discusses

---

9   Cynthia L. Ogden, PhD, Margaret D. Carroll, MSPH, Brian K. Kit, MD, MPH, Katherine M. Flegal, PhD. Prevalence of Childhood and Adult Obesity in the United States, 2011-2012, *JAMA*, 2014, 311 (8), 806-814. doi: 10:1001/jama2014.732.

10   Dr. Andrew Weil's Self-Healing 2014 Annual Edition, OneSource Content Marketing, LLC, 2015.

11   *Id.*

12   Sifferlin, Alexandra, The Weight Loss Trap: Why Your Diet Isn't Working, *Time*, May 25, 2017

the challenges to the metabolism posed by the process of calorie restriction also cited 2017 as the year that topped the charts on U.S. obesity levels.

Whether the correct figure is, in fact, roughly one-third of the U.S. population or two-thirds of the population, as a nation, we have cause for concern. In fact, the discrepancy in figures could be due to the fact that obesity seems to be on the rise, which was corroborated in other articles I have read. The *JAMA* study mentioned above, while reported in 2014, dates back to a study period of 2011-2012; whereas Dr. Weil's statistics, though reported in 2015, are from investigations done in 2014 and likely reflects the upward trend in obesity as compared to the *JAMA* study. The rates have only been rising and a solution is desperately needed.

Of course, we don't need medical journals to tell us this. As we all know, obesity is all too prevalent in our society.

The CDC's website, in discussing this problem, states that obesity-related conditions include heart disease, stroke, Type 2 diabetes, and certain types of cancer—some of the leading causes of preventable death. *The Times* article lists these and other maladies such as infertility, depression, and the number one cause of death beyond even cigarette smoking as casualties of obesity.[13]

The CDC further states on their website that medical costs for obesity-related conditions are tipping the scales, as well. According to their website, the estimated annual medical cost of obesity in the U.S. was $147 billion, with medical costs for those who are obese coming in at $1,429 higher than those of normal weight.[14]

---

13 *Id.*
14 The Center for Disease Control cites Eric A. Finkelstein, Justin G. Trogdon, Joel W. Cohen and William Dietz. Annual Medical Spending Attributable To Obesity: Payer-And Service-Specific Estimates. *Health Affairs*, 28, no. 5 (2009): w822-w831 (published online July 27, 2009; 10.1377/ hlthaff.28.5.w822)

Widespread obesity raised medical care costs by $315.8 billion in 2010, according to John Cawley, an economics professor at Cornell University in Ithaca, New York.[15] He agrees that obesity is a significant risk factor for diabetes, cardiovascular disease, and other life-threatening or life-shortening conditions.[16]

What Is Going On? Why Can't I Lose Weight?

Obesity is the product of a metabolism that does not burn off as many calories as the body consumes. So, what does almost every person do in an attempt to lose weight, what we have been taught to do and conditioned to believe before this remarkable discovery in food science? You guessed it: we restrict our calories, hoping to lose weight and shed the extra stored fat. But then one of two things happen: either we are too hungry to keep that up, or our bodies fear starvation and, as a result, slow down metabolism while also decreasing muscle mass; thus paving the way for later weight gain. In fact, the *Times* article that I mentioned above spoke about metabolisms decreasing their rate by a whopping 700 calories a day in response to drastic dieting.[17]

Before we go any further, let's first define "metabolism."

The Merriam-Webster dictionary defines "metabolism" as the sum of the processes in the buildup and destruction of protoplasm; specifically: the chemical changes in living cells by which energy is provided for vital processes and activities and new material is assimilated.

---

15 Cawley, J., et.al. Savings in Medical Expenditures Associated with Reductions in Body Mass Index Among US Adults with Obesity, by Diabetes Status. *Pharmacoeconomics*. www.ncbi.nlm.nih.gov/pubmed/25381647, 2015 Jul;33(7)707-22. Doi:10.1007/s40273-014-0230-2.

16 *Id.*

17 Sifferlin, Alexandra, *The Weight Loss Trap: Why Your Diet Isn't Working*, *Time*, May 25, 2017

As we can infer from this definition, if you are giving your body more energy (which is measured by the amount of kilocalories a food contains) than it uses for the vital processes and activities of your life, there will be a surplus. That surplus is stored for later use; usually as fat. While that might be great if one were living in the wilderness where food is scarce in the winter months, that is not our typical modern-day environment. Instead of burning off that excess fat during the cold winter months, we unfortunately just seem to pack on more pounds.

As was found in the Framingham Heart Study, an ongoing study of more than 10,000 people in Massachusetts (now considered one of the longest, most influential preventative and epidemiological research ever done), most adults will gain 20 pounds between the ages 25-55, if no steps are taken to avoid that gain.[18] What is peculiar here is that Framingham findings spurred a revolution in preventative care. Yet, even with the knowledge we have concerning obesity or being "just overweight," finding a lasting solution to weight gain continues to elude so many people.

Let's Turn That Around!

What most people don't know is that if you eat foods with a high thermogenic potential, you can turn that around. It's actually quite simple. I'll explain:

Thermogenesis is the process of heat production in organisms. By eating hot, you increase heat production in your body, thereby increasing your metabolism. So, instead of those extra kilocalories being transformed into fat to land in your belly, hips or thighs, they are burned off.

18 Dr. Andrew Weil's Self-Healing 2014 Annual Edition, OneSource Content Marketing, LLC, 2015.

Enter the Scene—
The Natural Metabolism Booster

Capsaicin is the *Star Ingredient* of EAT HOT...LOOK HOT. It's a huge part of what I call my secret sauce.

If you have never heard of this ingredient before, let me tell you a bit about it. There is a genus of flowering plants in the nightshade family called capsicums (commonly known as peppers[19]) that contain the bioactive ingredient capsaicin. Capsaicinoids are a group of chemicals which not only gives these plants and their fruits their fiery flavor, but also exert metabolic effects on those who consume them.

For starters, it is believed to double energy output for up to three hours after consumption. It may also work to decrease appetite centers in the brain by boosting the release of certain neurotransmitters. Plants belonging to this class are a hot ticket for revving up the metabolism. To benefit from this natural phenomenon, you will need to add red peppers, cayenne pepper, sriracha sauce (spicy or 'sweet and spicy'), jalapeños, habaneros, or tabasco sauce to the foods you eat. One study I came across showed weight loss with a non-spicy red bell pepper, which had a related compound to capsaicin called capsiate.

According to numerous reports in various peer-reviewed journals of physiology and science, the consumption of spicy food leads to greater thermogenesis and, in some cases, to greater satiety and satisfaction. The scientific studies cite capsaicin as a relevant example. Literature in various medical journals also discuss how these functional ingredients have the potential to produce significant effects on other metabolic targets beside satiety and thermogenesis (rate of metabolism), such as fat oxidation.

---

19 While they share the same colloquial name "pepper," and both cause burning sensations, there is no botanical relation between the table condiment pepper (black pepper, piper nigrum) and this plant.

It has also been shown that eating capsaicin-rich foods counteracts the typical bodily reaction of a slowing of the metabolism in response to weight loss.

How?

First, the active ingredient in the spicy fare, capsaicin, reduces your appetite so that you eat approximately 300 calories less at your current and next meal. Second, this same active ingredient revs up your metabolism so you burn extra calories that you wouldn't be burning otherwise. Peer-reviewed medical research shows that this metabolic rise occurs for 3–4 hours after consuming certain spices, roots (such as ginger), plants (tea, coffee) and peppers including one non-spicy pepper. And third, you increase what is called "lipid oxidation." What this means is that your body starts to break down fatty acids for the production of energy.

It's also not just what you eat, but when you eat it and how you eat it. For example, if you negate the hot part of the food you are consuming by rushing to drink, say, some milk or eating a piece of bread right away, you will also be diluting the benefit of the spice. I will discuss that in more detail in later chapters as I take you through Phases One through Four of the EAT HOT...LOOK HOT diet plan.

For now, just make a mental note that certain foods and drinks will, if consumed within the first few minutes of eating the capsaicin-rich foods, negate some of the effects of the hot spice. You can feel it right away in your mouth. The hot sensation will weaken. We will talk more about this later, and will cover strategies to resist this pitfall. For this reason, I recommend avoiding bread or milk products (except skim milk) right before and right after eating the spicy fare. Milk contains casein and this inactivates much of the capsaicin oil. To play it safe, avoid dairy 30 minutes before and after consuming anything with capsaicin if you want to burn fat and drop those extra pounds.

Capsiate, the ingredient in peppers which has much of the same structure as capsaicin, also promotes energy metabolism and suppresses body fat accumulation similarly to capsaicin, for a non-spicy alternative.[20] Non-users of spicy foods who wish to gain many of the weight reduction benefits gained from spicy peppers can eat sweet, non-pungent peppers rich in capsiate to aid in weight management efforts, though they won't experience the same weight loss factor as those who imbibe their meals and snacks with spicy foods.[21] If you absolutely can't acclimate to or tolerate spicy food, this is an alternative to get you Looking Hot.

Another study researched the anti-obesity effect of a capsicoside G-rich fraction (CRF) isolated from pepper seeds in diet-induced obese mice, finding that CRF could be used in a diet to help prevent obesity and obesity-related metabolic diseases.[22]

Bonus Tip:

Sprinkle a tiny dash of ground cayenne pepper (in powdered spice form) and a dash of cinnamon to your coffee, cappuccino, or latte. For a better blend of the spice, whip it up in the blender or steamer for 2 minutes and drink it before the spices settle on the top.

For even better weight-loss results, use a non-dairy milk alternative such as soy, almond, cashew, coconut or rice milk.

20 Ohnuki K, et al. Administration of capsiate, a non-pungent capsaicin analog, promotes energy metabolism and suppresses body fat accumulation in mice. *Biosci Biotechnol Biochem.* 2001 Dec;65(12):2735-40. https://www.ncbi.nlm.nih.gov/m/pubmed/11826971/?i=2&from=/22038945/related

21 Mary-Jon Ludy, et.al. The Effects of Capsaicin and Capsiate on Energy Balance: Critical Review and Meta-analyses of Studies in Humans. *Chem Senses.* 2012 Feb; 37(2): 103–121. https://www.ncbi.nlm.nih.gov/pmc/articles/PMC3257466/

22 Sung J., et.al. "Effect of the Capsicoside G-rich Fraction from Pepper (Capsicum annuum L.) Seeds on High-fat Diet-induced Obesity in Mice." *Phytother Res.* 2016 Nov;30(11):1848-1855. doi: 10.1002/ptr.5692. Epub 2016 Aug 19. https://www.ncbi.nlm.nih.gov/m/pubmed/27538894/?i=177&from=red%20pepper

As you have probably deduced by now, the secret sauce of the EAT HOT...LOOK HOT diet is full of peppers!

How Capsaicin Positively Affects Other Processes in the Body

Eating Hot has been shown to have positive effects on other bodily functions. Many of the research studies that I came across discuss at length the benefits of eating foods with capsaicin as their active ingredient for helping control blood sugar, for those suffering from Type 2 diabetes. In my research for this book, I have also come across scientific reviews showing its positive effects on inflammation (which experts agree contributes to all sorts of health conditions), in addition to other studies that show how capsaicin-containing foods fight viruses such as the common cold and flu. I go into greater details on the added health benefits of following EAT HOT... LOOK HOT in the *Full Edition*, for those who are interested in more in-depth discussions.

I would like to point out at the outset that it is not necessary to understand all the complex mechanisms at play if you find this kind of discussion overwhelming, confusing, or just plain tedious. The long and the short of it is simply that this diet plan results in easy weight loss. You will lose weight easily and quickly (if that's the speed you and your doctor choose), and you'll keep it off for as long as you continue to *Eat Hot*.

Adjusting the Diet Depending on Your Starting Point

You can adjust the amount of the key ingredients you'll be adding at some point(s) in your day to your own comfort zone, and go as slowly as you like. Some of you will see this as a sprint and others as a marathon. I've experienced it as both. The diet's phases are also somewhat subjective, meaning that if you are a person who is used to eating spicy food, you might need to add a little extra spice to the recipes noted for each phase of the diet. Conversely, if you are not used to eating any spicy food, you may need to reduce the pungency of the recipe suggestions until you have slowly built up a tolerance.

Don't forget to skip the bread and milk when you eat the spicy fare or you will dilute much of the capsaicin effect. If you love and must have your dairy at all times, pair the spicy fare with skim milk only for the best weight management effects.

The Beautiful Simplicity of EAT HOT...LOOK HOT

What is wonderful about EAT HOT...LOOK HOT is that it is all natural. No diet pills and nothing synthetic are involved—just the humble jalapeño and its related peppers.

It's a solution to the obesity problem that's made by God, not man.

The beauty of it lies in its simplicity.

CHAPTER FOUR

GETTING STARTED

Foods to Buy to Get Your Head-Start on
Looking Hot:

Chili Powder
Red Pepper Flakes
Jalapeños and Spicy Peppers
Jalapeño powder
Jalapeño Potato Chips
Cayenne Pepper
Ginger
Mustard
Tabasco Sauce
Salsa
Sriracha Sauce
Green Tea
Coffee
Black Pepper
Cumin
Coriander
Spicy Curries

More Bonus Recipes and *Eat Hot* Suggestions to Get You Started on the Path to *Look Hot:*

(Notice how simple they are and how easy it is to turn any meal into an EAT HOT...LOOK HOT drink, meal or snack!)

Spiced Hot Cocoa

Warm 7 ounces of soy (or other dairy-free milk alternative) in a pan for 2-3 minutes until warm but not boiling. Pour into a mug and add 2 tablespoons of pure cocoa powder. Then add a (tiny) dash of cayenne pepper powder for a spiced hot cocoa rich in polyphenols and capsaicin.

Spiced Ginger Soup

Buy any pre-made ginger soup that you like. Warm in a pan on the stove and add a pinch of cayenne pepper (plus a pinch of black pepper too in a few weeks' time)

Avocado Made Spicy

Cut an avocado into cubes. Add olive oil, salt and black pepper to taste. Add a pinch of cayenne pepper (start with about 1/20th of a teaspoon and work up from there). Stir.

Rice and/or Beans con Chili

Add Chili Powder to any rice and/or beans dish. Gradually increase amount of chili powder as you build your tolerance.

Potato Salad con Jalapeño (and Herring, if you choose)

Prepare or purchase your favorite potato salad.
Dice one jalapeño pepper, careful to remove all seeds and the veins. Add it to the potato salad. This dish tastes great with herring added in. Stir.

Spicy Meat Dishes Galore

Add cooked spicy peppers to the sauce of any meat dish, whether baked, cooked in a stew, boiled on the stovetop, or cooked in a crock pot. Go slow at first.
This simple incorporation can be adapted for chicken and lamb dishes too.

Meat-Based Soups with Spice

Add chili powder or cayenne pepper to any soup that is red meat-based. Go slow at first.
It will not taste good with chicken-based soups.

Tomato-Based Soups with Spice

Add chili powder or cayenne pepper to any tomato-based soup, particularly minestrone or cabbage soup. Go slow at first.
If there is red meat in there, or pasta, it will taste even better!

Indian Curry with Rice

By any Indian Curry that has chili powder or capsicum in it. If it has turmeric, ginger or black pepper too, even better! (The packaging should indicate how spicy the product is and be sure not to overdue it.) Warm. Pour it over prepared wild rice.

More Quick Bonus Tips to Get You Started on EAT HOT...LOOK HOT:

Phase One

- Add some chili pepper flakes, oregano, salt, a little bit of black pepper and a lot of olive oil to whole wheat linguini. (Optional add-ons for better taste: sautéed spinach and garlic)

- Add cheddar cheese, butter and chili powder to a mashed baked potato in its skin

- Add chili powder to meatloaf

- Chop and add some sweet peppers while sautéing potatoes

- Add cumin, black pepper, coriander and diced fresh garlic to your chicken soup as it cooks

- Add a dash of cayenne pepper to any meat- or tomato-based soup

Phase Two

- Pair tortillas or corn chips with spicy salsa

- Eat Jalapeño flavored chips, a handful at a time

- Add 1/8 teaspoon of cayenne pepper or chili powder to your scrambled eggs

- Add 1/8 teaspoon of cayenne pepper or chili powder to your hash-browns or sautéed potatoes

- Buy a bottle of *Sriracha Sauce* and dip baked salmon in it

- Bake chicken (with the skin on) in *Sriracha Sauce*

Phase Three

- Sprinkle a light coat of cayenne pepper on your favorite white fish before baking

- Sprinkle turmeric and red chili pepper flakes on lamb, chicken or beef kabobs

- Make your own *Spicy Mayo* by adding a hot *Sriracha Sauce* to mayonnaise. Use as a dip.

- Hold each bite of spicy food in your mouth for almost a full minute as you feel the heat intensify.

- Add cayenne pepper more liberally in your meat- or tomato-based soups

Phase Four

Instructions: Look at the call-out box right before the bonus recipe section that tells you what to buy at your next trip to the supermarket. Next: combine any of those listed non-pepper ingredients with the any of the hot pepper ingredients. For example, drink warm green tea with any Phase One, Two, or Three meal or snack. Or drink warm ginger tea. Alternatively, add mustard to one of the previous recipes. Add cayenne to your coffee. Add black pepper to the already spicy meals and snacks you prepare. Just sprinkle it in. The more frequently you add these 'additions' to your existing food and drink, and particularly together with the capsaicin-loaded foods, the more you will lose! Prepare to eat and look hot, hot and hotter!

These are just some quick suggestions off the top of my head to get you thinking in the *Hot* direction...

Don't forget that gradual incorporation of the *Hot Foods* is a very important component of the diet. It's also an important safety feature so when in doubt, please air on the side of caution. That's why I separate this diet into four phases. Don't forget to ask your doctor to weigh in on how spicy you can take this diet and to address any other health concerns that you may have, especially if you have Reflux Disease or are prone to ulcers.[23]

23   Per my interview with Jonathan Aviv, MD, FACS and author of *The Acid Watcher Diet*.

Dear Reader,

As you know, this book is only the abbreviated *Sneak Preview Edition* of EAT HOT...LOOK HOT, which is still in the recipe-gathering phase of production. I am working hard to bring you the full edition as soon as possible. However, I want to get the word out now, to essentially tell people that help is on the way and to start changing peoples' mindsets from one of hopelessness to one of hope for long-lasting, easy weight loss. I also want to introduce you to this ground-breaking weight loss/maintenance method, so you can not only mentally prepare yourself for success and *looking hot* but also actually get a head start! I hope that reading the opening chapters of the book did just that—if not, read on; because you are about to get an additional sneak preview into the forthcoming chapters of the full book.

Since you have already invested your valuable time and energy into reading the introductory chapters of EAT HOT...LOOK HOT, you can be amongst the first to receive the first printing of the full book. Simply sign up at *www.EatHotLookHotDiet.com* and my team will send you a periodic update of the book's progress, bonus tips, "Cooking Hot" videos, and other great content. Best of all, you will be the first to know about the full book's release, any option to pre-order it from Amazon.com, and our upcoming media appearances.

Even though the book is not finished yet, I am excited to share with you some of what I have already put together for you for the full book, EAT HOT...LOOK HOT, which will be released soon.

To hold you over in the meantime, here are the rest of the contents. And, I have a 21st-century secret to share with my dear readers: there will be lots of video clips, tutorials, and demos (with me and with world-class chefs) embedded within the book that can be accessed via scanning QR codes or simple clicks in the eBook version of EAT HOT...LOOK HOT.

Here are the topics covered in the forthcoming chapters.[24] I am also happy to include some of the key lessons you will take away from each chapter. Again: sign up now at www.EatHotLookHotDiet. com to be amongst the first to find out about the full book's release, get access to promotions and sales (and possibly pre-orders), plus get free bonus materials along the way by simply telling us where to send it to.

As promised, here is your sneak preview:

Chapter Four—Capsaicin: The Star Component in Scientific Studies into Weight Loss

Scientific Studies Back Up EAT HOT...LOOK HOT

We covered some basic science in Chapter Three, but wait—there's more ... much more!

In this chapter, you'll learn:

- How to boost your metabolism by eating certain spicy foods, and I'll tell you which

- What's really in a chili pepper and how it will help you to look your absolute best!

- When you *Eat Hot*, you'll naturally *Eat Less*

- Should you ingest capsaicin via pill or other forms?

- How much capsaicin is necessary?

---

24   Subject to change, as the book is being edited.

- How to attain a synergistic effect, where 1 + 1 = more than two
- How Amy got out of her "Catch-22," where each time she shed those extra pounds, her metabolism slowed down in response
- How to achieve fat-busting results
- The importance of building up tolerance and not over-doing it
- A shortcut to getting your endorphins flowing
- Why capsaicin may be the next anti-obesity drug
- Why EAT HOT…LOOK HOT is *The Diet* to end all other diets

Chapter Five—Hands on the Peppers

- First things first—safety in handling the peppers
- What makes dried pepper hot

Chapter Six—An Overview of the Four Phases of EAT HOT…LOOK HOT

- What you can expect from this diet plan
- Fundamentals of the diet
- Understanding how heat is measured in spices and food
- Heat is in the eye (or, really, the taste buds) of the beholder. Where do you fit on the spectrum?

Chapter Seven—Getting Started, Getting Slim

- Here we begin Phase One of EAT HOT…LOOK HOT
- How to adjust the diet to your own pace
- Simple adaptations you can make to your current meals and snacks to call it a weight-loss day!
- Easy recipes for Phase One meals and snacks
- Practical alternatives to cooking

- A practical guide to supermarket products that we identify as Phase One products

- A table of popular peppers and their approximate Scoville Heat Index. Some are way hotter than others!

- Recipes from some of Miami's best restaurant and hotel chefs, adapted to Phase One of EAT HOT...LOOK HOT

Chapter Eight—Taking it to the Next Hot Level

- Here we begin Phase Two of EAT HOT...LOOK HOT

- Simple adaptations you can make to your current meals and snacks to call it a weight-loss day!

- Easy recipes for Phase Two meals and snacks

- A practical guide to supermarket products that we identify as Phase Two products, no need to cook anything if you don't like to cook. Don't worry: I have it all mapped out for you with product guides.

- Practical alternatives to cooking

- Recipes from some of Miami's best restaurant and hotel chefs, adapted to Phase Two of EAT HOT...LOOK HOT

Chapter Nine—Feeling Hot, Hot, Hot

- Here we begin Phase Three of *EAT HOT...LOOK HOT*

- Simple adaptations you can make to your current meals and snacks to add Phase 3 hotness into your weight-loss day!

- Easy recipes for Phase Three meals and snacks

- A practical guide to Phase Three supermarket products

- Practical alternatives to cooking at home

- Easy tips to intensify the heat of any bite or sip

- Recipes from some of Miami's best restaurant and hotel chefs, adapted to Phase Three of EAT HOT...LOOK HOT

Chapter Ten—Eating Hotter, Looking Hotter

- This is a "surprise chapter"

- Here we begin Phase Four of EAT HOT...LOOK HOT— and it is not what you expect it to be

- Synergistic food combinations—what to add into your meals and snacks to look even hotter!

- Additional adaptations you can make to your current meals and snacks to keep the fat-busting going all day and all night (if you do it right)

- Easy recipes for Phase Four meals and snacks

- A practical guide to supermarket products that we identify as Phase Four /very hot products

- Practical alternatives to cooking

- What constitutes too much spice?

- Recipes from some of Miami's best restaurant and hotel chefs, adapted to Phase Four of EAT HOT...LOOK HOT

Chapter Eleven—EAT HOT...LOOK HOT
Health Benefits beyond Weight Loss

- Capsaicin's health benefits beyond weight management

- A nutritional breakdown of some chili peppers

- Pain control

- Cardiovascular benefits

- *Should ulcer sufferers avoid spicy food?*

- Research update: Cayenne pepper contributes to longevity

- Research update: How Cayenne pepper combats hair loss

- Research update: How Cayenne pepper provides extra stamina

- Research update: How Cayenne helps with blood circulation

- Many more research updates

- Extra benefits to diabetics

- *Salsa, anyone?* Studies point to protection against pathogens.

Chapter Twelve—EAT HOT...LOOK HOT
Gives a Natural Glow

- It won't just be your body that looks great. Your skin will glow, too, if you follow the EAT HOT...LOOK HOT plan

Chapter Thirteen—Men Get Hotter Too!

- Additional sexual enhancement benefits for men (or the man in your life, if you feed him certain spicy foods)

- Better blood flow all-around is better for the bedroom too! After reading this chapter, ask your physician if you can try this in lieu of Viagra.

- Link between consuming capsaicin-loaded food and higher levels of testosterone

- Better stamina for performance, studies show. Feel like your younger self all over again…

Chapter Fourteen—Mindful Eating

- How EAT HOT...LOOK HOT re-calibrates your brain's hunger signals

- How EAT HOT...LOOK HOT stops binge-eating

- Mindful Eating becomes second-nature because you are urged to keep the spicy fare in your mouth longer than usual to amplify its fat-busing effects. This ties in with mindfulness-based meditation practice, which in turn helps the brain become more sensitive to feelings of satiety and hunger

- Mindful Eating confers its own separate health benefits, as well.

Chapter Fifteen—Bonus Recipes from Miami's Top Chefs

- All recipes are adaptable to Phases One through Four

Chapter Sixteen—Success Stories

- One day, this could be you!

Final Note
Appendix A—Footnotes and References
Appendix B—Recipe Index

And there you have it…Almost.

Can't wait for the full book to come out? Neither can we.

Simply go to www.EatHotLookHotDiet.com, sign up, and stay in the know or submit your results.

If you would like to become an Ambassador or get more involved in this *Hot Sensation*, send us your success story via the website by clicking on "I'm a Success Story" (if not readily apparent, click the drop-down bar.) Help spread the word to your friends and contacts on social media if this works for you, which I expect it will.

You can also do a service to others by leaving a review of EAT HOT…LOOK HOT *Sneak Preview Edition* on Amazon.com, Goodreads.com or other book-buying (or reading) sites as people rely on feedback from other readers like you. All reviews are greatly appreciated!

Wishing you hotness, health, and dreams coming true

-Alessandra

Made in the USA
Lexington, KY
02 January 2018